IPL Age-Defying

Age-Defying Beauty: The Science Behind IPL Treatments for Women 40+

Michelle Lopez Lopez

Table Of Contents

Chapter 1: Understanding IPL Treatments 3

What is IPL? 3

How does IPL work? 4

Bene ts of IPL treatments for aging skin 5

Chapter 2: Common Skin Concerns for Women 40+ 6

Fine lines and wrinkles 6

Age spots and sun damage 8

Uneven skin tone 9

Chapter 3: The Science Behind IPL Treatments 10

How IPL targets pigmentation 11

Stimulating collagen production with IPL 12

Improving skin texture with IPL 13

Chapter 4: Preparing for an IPL Treatment 14

Consultation with a dermatologist 14

Skin care regimen before treatment 16

What to expect during the treatment 17

Chapter 5: Post-Treatment Care and Maintenance 18

Managing side effects of IPL 18

Protecting your skin after treatment 20

Long-term bene ts of regular IPL treatments 21

Chapter 6: Real Women, Real Results 23

Testimonials from women who have tried IPL treatments

Before and after photos of IPL treatments for aging skin   24

Chapter 7: FAQs about IPL Treatments for Women 40+   **26**

Is IPL safe for aging skin?   26

How many treatments are needed for optimal results?   27

Can IPL treatments be combined with other skin care procedures?   28

Chapter 8: Finding the Right IPL Provider   **30**

Questions to ask when choosing an IPL provider   30

Researching the credentials and experience of IPL practitioners   31

Cost considerations for IPL treatments   32

Chapter 9: Embracing Age-Defying Beauty with IPL   **34**

The psychological bene ts of looking and feeling younger   34

Maintaining con dence and self-esteem as you age   35

Embracing the aging process with grace and positivity   36

Chapter 1: Understanding IPL Treatments
What is IPL?

Intense pulsed light (IPL) is a popular and e ective treatment for various skin concerns, particularly for women in the 40+ age group. IPL uses pulses of light to target speci c skin issues such as sun damage, age spots, redness, and ne lines. Unlike laser treatments that use a single wavelength of light, IPL uses multiple wavelengths, making it versatile and suitable for a wide range of skin types and conditions.

IPL works by delivering pulses of light energy to the deeper layers of the skin, stimulating the production of collagen and elastin. This results in improved skin texture, rmness, and overall rejuvenation. IPL treatments are non-invasive and require little to no downtime, making them a convenient option for busy women looking to address signs of aging and sun damage without undergoing surgery or lengthy recovery periods.

One of the key bene ts of IPL is its ability to target multiple skin concerns in a single treatment session. Whether you're looking to reduce the appearance of age spots, minimize ne lines, or improve overall skin tone and texture, IPL can help you achieve your desired results. With regular IPL treatments, women in the 40+ age group can enjoy smoother, more youthful-looking skin that radiates health and v it alit y.

It's important to note that IPL treatments should be performed by a quali ed and experienced skincare professional to ensure safety and optimal results. During your initial consultation, your skincare provider will assess your skin type and concerns, develop a customized treatment plan, and discuss what to expect during and after your IPL sessions. With proper care and maintenance, IPL can be a valuable tool in your anti-aging skincare routine, helping you maintain a youthful and radiant complexion well into your 40s and beyond.

In conclusion, IPL is a safe, e ective, and non-invasive treatment option for women in the 40+ age group looking to rejuvenate their skin and address common signs of aging. By targeting multiple skin concerns in a single session and stimulating collagen production, IPL can help you achieve smoother, more youthful-looking skin with minimal downtime. With the guidance of a skilled skincare professional, IPL can be a valuable addition to your anti-aging skincare routine, helping you maintain a radiant and age-defying complexion for years to come.

How does IPL work?

As women age, they may start to notice changes in their skin such as sun spots, wrinkles, and uneven pigmentation. Intense pulsed light (IPL) treatments have become a popular option for women age 40+ looking to rejuvenate their skin and achieve a more youthful appearance. But how exactly does IPL work?

IPL works by delivering high-intensity pulses of light to the skin, targeting speci c pigments such as melanin and hemoglobin. This light energy is absorbed by the pigment in the skin, causing it to break down and fade over time. IPL treatments can e ectively reduce the appearance of sun spots, freckles, and redness, giving the skin a more even tone and texture.

One of the key bene ts of IPL treatments is that they are non-invasive and require minimal downtime. Unlike more aggressive procedures like laser resurfacing, IPL treatments are gentle on the skin and do not require anesthesia. Patients can typically resume their normal activities immediately after treatment, making it a convenient option for busy women in their 40s and beyond.

Another important aspect of how IPL works is its ability to stimulate collagen production in the skin. Collagen is a protein that gives skin its rmness and elasticity, but production naturally decreases with age. By stimulating collagen production, IPL treatments can help improve skin texture, reduce ne lines and wrinkles, and give the skin a more youthful appearance.

In conclusion, IPL treatments are a safe and e ective option for women age 40+ looking to rejuvenate their skin and achieve a more youthful appearance. By targeting speci c pigments in the skin and stimulating collagen production, IPL treatments can help reduce the appearance of sun spots, wrinkles, and uneven pigmentation. With minimal downtime and impressive results, IPL is a popular choice for women looking to defy the signs of aging and maintain a radiant complexion.

Benefits of IPL treatments for aging skin

As we age, our skin undergoes numerous changes, including the development of ne lines, wrinkles, and age spots. Fortunately, Intense Pulsed Light (IPL) treatments o er a non-invasive solution to combat these common signs of aging. In this subchapter, we will explore the various bene ts of IPL treatments for aging skin, speci cally tailored to women in the 40+ age group.

One of the key bene ts of IPL treatments for aging skin is their ability to target multiple skin concerns at once. IPL technology works by delivering pulses of light energy to the deeper layers of the skin, stimulating collagen production and improving overall skin tone and texture. This can help to reduce the appearance of ne lines, wrinkles, and age spots, giving the skin a more youthful and radiant appearance.

In addition to addressing visible signs of aging, IPL treatments can also help to improve the overall health of the skin. By stimulating collagen production, IPL treatments can help to strengthen the skin's structure and improve its ability to retain moisture. This can result in rmer, more hydrated skin that is better able to resist the e ects of aging and environmental damage.

Another bene t of IPL treatments for aging skin is their non-invasive nature. Unlike more aggressive treatments such as chemical peels or laser resurfacing, IPL treatments are gentle on the skin and require minimal downtime. This makes them a convenient option for women in the 40+ age group who may not have the time or desire to undergo more intensive procedures.

Finally, IPL treatments are safe and e ective for women of all skin types. Whether you have fair skin or a darker complexion, IPL technology can be customized to suit your speci c needs and address your unique skin concerns. This makes IPL treatments a versatile and inclusive option for women looking to rejuvenate their skin and regain a more youthful appearance.

Chapter 2: Common Skin Concerns for Women 40+

Fine lines and wrinkles

As we age, ne lines and wrinkles become more prominent on our skin, leading many women in the 40+ age group to seek out e ective treatments to combat these signs of aging. One popular option that has gained traction in recent years is Intense Pulsed Light (IPL) therapy. IPL treatments utilize high-intensity pulses of light to target areas of pigmentation, vascular imperfections, and ne lines on the skin, resulting in a more youthful and radiant complexion.

Fine lines and wrinkles are a natural part of the aging process, but that doesn't mean we have to accept them as inevitable. IPL treatments can help to reduce the appearance of ne lines and wrinkles by stimulating collagen production in the skin. Collagen is a protein that gives skin its structure and elasticity, and as we age, our bodies produce less of it. By increasing collagen production through IPL therapy, we can help to plump up the skin and smooth out ne lines and wrinkles.

One of the key bene ts of IPL treatments for ne lines and wrinkles is that they are non-invasive and require minimal downtime. Unlike more aggressive treatments like chemical peels or laser resurfacing, IPL therapy is gentle on the skin and typically only causes mild redness or swelling that subsides within a few hours. This makes IPL treatments an attractive option for women in the 40+ age group who want to improve the appearance of their skin without undergoing more invasive procedures.

In addition to reducing the appearance of ne lines and wrinkles, IPL treatments can also help to improve overall skin tone and texture. The high-intensity pulses of light used in IPL therapy can target areas of hyperpigmentation, sun damage, and redness, resulting in a more even complexion. By addressing multiple skin concerns in one treatment, IPL therapy can help women in the 40+ age group achieve a more youthful and radiant appearance.

In conclusion, ne lines and wrinkles are a common concern for women in the 40+ age group, but they don't have to be a permanent xture on our skin. IPL treatments o er a safe and e ective solution for reducing the appearance of ne lines and wrinkles, while also improving overall skin tone and texture. If you're looking to turn back the clock and achieve a more youthful complexion, consider incorporating IPL therapy into your skincare routine. With regular treatments, you can enjoy smoother, rmer, and more radiant skin well into your 40s and beyond.

Age spots and sun damage

Age spots and sun damage are common concerns for women in the 40+ age group. These dark spots, often referred to as "liver spots" or "sun spots," are caused by prolonged exposure to the sun's harmful UV rays. Over time, these spots can become more pronounced and can make the skin appear dull and aged. Fortunately, there are e ective treatments available, such as Intense Pulsed Light (IPL) therapy, that can help reduce the appearance of age spots and sun damage.

IPL therapy works by using high-intensity pulses of light to target the melanin in the skin, which is responsible for dark spots. The light energy is absorbed by the melanin, causing it to break down and fade over time. This results in a more even skin tone and a reduction in the appearance of age spots. IPL treatments are non-invasive and require little to no downtime, making them a convenient option for women in the 40+ age group who are looking to improve the appearance of their skin.

In addition to targeting age spots, IPL therapy can also help reduce the signs of sun damage on the skin. Sun damage, such as ne lines, wrinkles, and uneven skin texture, can be improved with IPL treatments. The light energy stimulates collagen production in the skin, which can help improve skin elasticity and rmness. This can result in a more youthful and radiant complexion for women in the 40+ age group.

It is important for women in the 40+ age group to protect their skin from further damage by wearing sunscreen daily and avoiding prolonged sun exposure. However, for those who already have signs of age spots and sun damage, IPL therapy can be a highly e ective solution. With a series of treatments, women can see signi cant improvements in the appearance of their skin, leading to a more youthful and vibrant complexion.

In conclusion, age spots and sun damage are common concerns for women in the 40+ age group, but there are e ective treatments available, such as IPL therapy, that can help reduce the appearance of these issues. By targeting the melanin in the skin, IPL treatments can fade age spots and improve skin tone, while also stimulating collagen production to reduce the signs of sun damage. With proper skin care and regular IPL treatments, women in the 40+ age group can achieve a more youthful and radiant complexion.

Uneven skin tone

Uneven skin tone is a common concern among women in the 40+ age group. As we age, our skin can become discolored due to a variety of factors, including sun damage, hormonal changes, and genetics. Uneven skin tone can manifest as dark spots, redness, or sallowness, and can make us look older than we feel. Fortunately, there are e ective treatments available to help improve the appearance of uneven skin tone, including Intense Pulsed Light (IPL) therapy.

IPL treatments work by delivering pulses of light energy to the skin, targeting pigment cells and causing them to break down and fade away. This can help to reduce the appearance of dark spots and redness, resulting in a more even skin tone. IPL treatments are safe and non-invasive, making them a popular choice for women looking to improve the appearance of their skin without undergoing surgery or harsh chemical peels.

In addition to improving the appearance of uneven skin tone, IPL treatments can also help to stimulate collagen production in the skin. Collagen is a protein that helps to keep our skin rm and elastic, but levels of collagen naturally decrease as we age. By stimulating collagen production, IPL treatments can help to improve the overall texture and quality of the skin, resulting in a more youthful and radiant complexion.

It is important to note that IPL treatments are not a one-size- ts-all solution for uneven skin tone. Di erent skin types and concerns may require di erent treatment protocols, so it is important to consult with a skincare professional before undergoing IPL therapy. Additionally, it is important to protect your skin from further damage by wearing sunscreen and avoiding excessive sun exposure.

Overall, IPL treatments can be a highly e ective solution for women in the 40+ age group looking to improve the appearance of uneven skin tone. By targeting pigment cells and stimulating collagen production, IPL therapy can help to reduce the appearance of dark spots, redness, and sallowness, resulting in a more even and youthful complexion. Consult with a skincare professional to determine if IPL treatments are right for you and to develop a personalized treatment plan.

Chapter 3: The Science Behind IPL Treatments

How IPL targets pigmentation

Intense Pulsed Light (IPL) has become a popular treatment for targeting pigmentation issues in women over the age of 40. IPL works by emitting high-intensity pulses of light that penetrate the skin and target melanin, the pigment responsible for dark spots and uneven skin tone. This non-invasive treatment is a safe and e ective way to reduce the appearance of pigmentation and achieve a more youthful complexion.

One of the ways IPL targets pigmentation is by heating up the melanin in the skin, causing it to break up and disperse. This process helps to fade dark spots and even out skin tone over time. IPL can also stimulate collagen production, which can improve the overall texture and rmness of the skin, further reducing the appearance of pigmentation.

Another way IPL targets pigmentation is by targeting blood vessels in the skin that may be contributing to redness or discoloration. By constricting these blood vessels, IPL can help to reduce redness and create a more even skin tone. This can be particularly bene cial for women who struggle with rosacea or other vascular skin conditions.

IPL treatments are typically done in a series of sessions, spaced several weeks apart. This allows the skin to heal and regenerate between treatments, leading to gradual but noticeable improvements in pigmentation issues. Most women see signi cant results after just a few sessions, with continued improvement over time.

Overall, IPL is a versatile and e ective treatment for targeting pigmentation in women over the age of 40. By harnessing the power of light energy to break up melanin and target blood vessels, IPL can help women achieve a more youthful and radiant complexion. If you struggle with pigmentation concerns, consider scheduling a consultation with a quali ed IPL provider to see if this treatment is right for you.

Stimulating collagen production with IPL

As we age, our skin naturally loses collagen, leading to the formation of ne lines, wrinkles, and sagging. Intense pulsed light (IPL) treatments have been shown to stimulate collagen production in the skin, helping to reverse these signs of aging and restore a more youthful appearance. In this subchapter, we will explore how IPL works to stimulate collagen production and the bene ts it can o er women in the 40+ age group.

Collagen is a protein that provides structure and elasticity to the skin, helping it to maintain its rmness and smoothness. As we age, our bodies produce less collagen, leading to the formation of wrinkles and sagging skin. IPL treatments work by delivering pulses of light energy to the skin, which penetrates the dermis and stimulates the production of new collagen. This helps to tighten and rm the skin, reducing the appearance of ne lines and wrinkles.

One of the key bene ts of IPL treatments for stimulating collagen production is that they are non-invasive and require no downtime. Unlike surgical procedures that can be painful and require weeks of recovery time, IPL treatments are quick and relatively painless, with most patients experiencing only mild discomfort during the procedure. This makes IPL an attractive option for women in the 40+ age group who want to improve the appearance of their skin without undergoing surgery.

In addition to stimulating collagen production, IPL treatments can also help to improve the overall texture and tone of the skin. The light energy used in IPL treatments can target pigmentation issues, such as sun spots and age spots, helping to even out the skin tone and create a more youthful appearance. IPL can also help to reduce the appearance of broken capillaries and redness, giving the skin a more radiant and healthy glow.

Overall, IPL treatments can be a highly e ective way for women in the 40+ age group to stimulate collagen production and achieve a more youthful appearance. By targeting the underlying causes of aging skin, such as collagen loss and pigmentation issues, IPL treatments can help to improve the texture, tone, and rmness of the skin, giving women a renewed sense of con dence and beauty. If you are looking to turn back the clock and rejuvenate your skin, consider exploring the bene ts of IPL treatments for age-defying beauty.

Improving skin texture with IPL

As we age, many of us begin to notice changes in our skin texture. Fine lines, wrinkles, and uneven skin tone can all contribute to a dull and aged appearance. Fortunately, there are treatments available to help improve skin texture and achieve a more youthful complexion. One such treatment is Intense Pulsed Light (IPL) therapy, which has been shown to be e ective in reducing the signs of aging and improving overall skin texture.

IPL works by delivering high-energy light pulses to the skin, targeting speci c areas of concern such as sun damage, age spots, and redness. These pulses penetrate the skin and stimulate collagen production, which helps to improve skin texture and reduce the appearance of ne lines and wrinkles. IPL treatments are non-invasive and require little to no downtime, making them a popular choice for women looking to rejuvenate their skin.

One of the key bene ts of IPL therapy is its ability to target multiple skin concerns at once. Whether you are dealing with sun damage, age spots, or redness, IPL can help to improve overall skin texture and tone. By stimulating collagen production, IPL treatments can also help to plump up the skin and reduce the appearance of ne lines and wrinkles, giving you a more youthful and radiant complexion.

In addition to improving skin texture, IPL therapy can also help to reduce the appearance of acne scars and other blemishes. By targeting the underlying causes of these skin concerns, IPL treatments can help to smooth out the skin and improve its overall texture. This can be especially bene cial for women in their 40s and beyond who may be dealing with the lingering e ects of acne from their younger years.

Overall, IPL therapy is a safe and e ective way to improve skin texture and achieve a more youthful complexion. Whether you are dealing with sun damage, age spots, or ne lines and wrinkles, IPL treatments can help to rejuvenate your skin and restore a more youthful appearance. If you are a woman
in your 40s or older looking to improve your skin texture, consider scheduling an IPL treatment to experience the bene ts for yourself.

Chapter 4: Preparing for an IPL Treatment
Consultation with a dermatologist

As we age, our skin goes through many changes that can leave us feeling less con dent about our appearance. One of the most common concerns for women in their 40s is the development of age spots, ne lines, and wrinkles. Fortunately, there are advanced treatments available to help combat these signs of aging, such as Intense Pulsed Light (IPL) therapy. If you are considering IPL treatments, it is important to consult with a dermatologist rst to ensure that it is the right option for you. Consulting with a dermatologist before undergoing IPL treatments is essential because they can assess your skin type, concerns, and overall health to determine if you are a suitable candidate for this type of therapy. They can also provide valuable information about what to expect during the treatment process, any potential side e ects, and how to properly care for your skin post-treatment. Additionally, a dermatologist can customize a treatment plan that is tailored to your speci c needs and goals.

During your consultation with a dermatologist, be sure to discuss any medications you are currently taking, as well as any medical conditions you may have. This information will help your dermatologist determine the best approach for your IPL treatments and minimize the risk of any adverse reactions. It is also important to communicate your desired outcomes and any concerns you may have about the procedure with your dermatologist so they can address them accordingly.

Furthermore, consulting with a dermatologist will allow you to ask any questions you may have about IPL treatments and gain a better understanding of how they work. Your dermatologist can explain the science behind IPL therapy and provide you with realistic expectations about the results you can achieve. They can also recommend additional skincare products or treatments that can complement your IPL sessions and help you maintain healthy, youthful-looking skin.

In conclusion, consulting with a dermatologist before undergoing IPL treatments is a crucial step in the process of achieving age-defying beauty. Their expertise and guidance will ensure that you receive safe and e ective treatment that is tailored to your individual needs. By taking the time to consult with a dermatologist, you can feel con dent in your decision to pursue IPL therapy and take proactive steps towards maintaining radiant, youthful skin well into your 40s and beyond.

Skin care regimen before treatment

As women age, taking care of their skin becomes increasingly important, especially before undergoing any kind of treatment like Intense Pulsed Light (IPL). A proper skin care regimen before treatment can not only enhance the e ectiveness of the treatment but also ensure better results in the long run. In this subchapter, we will discuss the essential steps that women in the age group of 40+ should follow to prepare their skin for IPL treatments.

The rst step in any skin care regimen before treatment is to cleanse the skin thoroughly. Use a gentle cleanser that is suitable for your skin type to remove dirt, oil, and makeup from the skin's surface. This will help the IPL treatment penetrate more e ectively and prevent any blockages that could hinder the results.

After cleansing, it is important to exfoliate the skin to remove dead skin cells and unclog pores. Exfoliation can be done using chemical exfoliants like AHAs or BHAs or physical exfoliants like scrubs. This step will help improve the skin's texture and allow the IPL treatment to target the deeper layers of the skin more e ectively.

Moisturizing is another crucial step in preparing your skin for IPL treatments. Use a hydrating moisturizer that is suitable for your skin type to keep your skin hydrated and plump. This will not only improve the results of the IPL treatment but also help in reducing any potential side e ects like dryness or irritation.

In addition to cleansing, exfoliating, and moisturizing, it is important to protect your skin from the sun before undergoing IPL treatments. UV exposure can not only damage the skin but also interfere with the results of the treatment. Make sure to use a broad-spectrum sunscreen with an SPF of 30 or higher every day, even if you are not planning to be outdoors for long periods.

Lastly, it is recommended to avoid any harsh skincare products or treatments in the weeks leading up to your IPL treatment. This includes things like chemical peels, laser treatments, or strong exfoliants. These can make your skin more sensitive and increase the risk of adverse reactions during the IPL treatment. Stick to a gentle and consistent skincare routine to ensure the best possible outcome from your IPL treatment.

What to expect during the treatment

As women age, many may begin to notice changes in their skin such as ne lines, wrinkles, and age spots. Intense pulsed light (IPL) treatments have become a popular option for those looking to combat these signs of aging. In this subchapter, we will discuss what women in the 40+ age group can expect during IPL treatments.

During an IPL treatment, a handheld device is used to deliver pulses of light to the skin. This light is absorbed by the pigment in the skin, causing the blood vessels and collagen beneath the skin to constrict. This can help to reduce redness, improve the texture of the skin, and stimulate the production of new collagen.

Before beginning an IPL treatment, it is important to schedule a consultation with a quali ed provider. During this consultation, the provider will assess the skin and determine if IPL is the best option for the individual. They will also discuss the expected results, any potential risks or side e ects, and the number of treatments that may be needed.

Women undergoing IPL treatments can expect to feel a mild snapping or stinging sensation during the procedure. Some may experience redness, swelling, or darkening of the treated areas immediately following the treatment, but these side e ects typically subside within a few hours to a few days. It is important to follow the post-treatment care instructions provided by the provider to minimize any discomfort and ensure optimal results.

Results from IPL treatments are not immediate and may take several weeks to become noticeable. Most women will require a series of treatments spaced a few weeks apart to achieve the desired results. IPL treatments can help to improve the overall appearance of the skin, reducing the signs of aging and giving women in the 40+ age group a more youthful and radiant complexion.

Chapter 5: Post-Treatment Care and Maintenance

Managing side effects of IPL

Managing side e ects of IPL treatments is an important aspect of ensuring a successful and comfortable experience for women in the 40+ age group. While IPL treatments can provide signi cant bene ts in rejuvenating the skin and reducing signs of aging, it is not uncommon for patients to experience some side e ects following the procedure. By understanding how to e ectively manage these side e ects, women can maximize the bene ts of their IPL treatments and minimize any discomfort or co mp licat io n s .

One common side e ect of IPL treatments is redness and swelling in the treated area. This is a normal response to the light energy used in the procedure, and typically subsides within a few hours to a few days. To help minimize redness and swelling, women can apply a cool compress to the treated area and avoid hot showers or excessive heat exposure. Additionally, using gentle skincare products and avoiding harsh chemicals or exfoliants can help to soothe the skin and promote healing.

Another potential side e ect of IPL treatments is temporary pigmentation changes, such as darkening or lightening of the skin. While these changes are usually mild and resolve on their own over time, women can help to expedite the process by using sunscreen consistently and avoiding sun exposure. In some cases, topical treatments or creams may be recommended by a skincare professional to help fade any pigmentation changes and restore an even skin tone.

It is also important for women undergoing IPL treatments to be aware of the risk of blistering or crusting in the treated area. While these side e ects are less common, they can occur if the skin is not properly cared for following the procedure. To prevent blistering or crusting, women should avoid picking or scratching at the treated area and follow any post-treatment instructions provided by their skincare professional. Keeping the skin moisturized and protected can also help to prevent these side e ects from occurring.

In addition to physical side e ects, some women may also experience emotional or psychological side e ects following IPL treatments. It is not uncommon for women to feel self-conscious or anxious about their appearance during the healing process, especially if there are visible side e ects such as redness or pigmentation changes. Seeking support from friends, family, or a mental health professional can help women to navigate these feelings and feel more con dent in their decision to undergo IPL treatments. Remember, the bene ts of IPL treatments often outweigh any temporary side e ects, and with proper care and management, women can achieve beautiful, age-defying results that enhance their natural beauty.

Protecting your skin after treatment

After undergoing IPL treatments, it is crucial to protect your skin to maintain the results and prevent potential damage. Here are some tips to help you care for your skin post-treatment.

Firstly, it is important to avoid direct sun exposure for at least a week after your IPL treatment. The intense pulsed light can make your skin more sensitive to the sun's harmful rays, increasing the risk of sunburn and hyperpigmentation. Make sure to wear a broad-spectrum sunscreen with an SPF of at least 30 whenever you go outside, even on cloudy days.

Secondly, moisturizing is key to keeping your skin hydrated and promoting healing after IPL treatments. Use a gentle, non-comedogenic moisturizer to soothe any redness or irritation and prevent dryness. Look for products that contain ingredients like hyaluronic acid, glycerin, and ceramides to lock in moisture and restore your skin's barrier.

In addition to sunscreen and moisturizer, it is also important to avoid harsh skincare products that can irritate your skin post-IPL treatment. Stay away from products containing retinoids, exfoliating acids, and fragrances, as they can cause further sensitivity and redness. Stick to gentle cleansers and serums that are speci cally formulated for sensitive skin to prevent any adverse reactions.

Furthermore, staying hydrated and maintaining a healthy diet can also promote skin healing and prevent any complications after IPL treatments. Drink plenty of water to keep your skin hydrated from the inside out, and incorporate foods rich in antioxidants, vitamins, and minerals to support your skin's recovery process. Avoid alcohol and ca eine, as they can dehydrate your skin and hinder the healing process.

By following these post-treatment skincare tips, you can protect your skin and maintain the results of your IPL treatments for a more youthful and radiant complexion. Remember to consult with your skincare specialist for personalized recommendations and guidance on how to care for your skin after undergoing IPL treatments.

As women reach the age of 40 and beyond, they may start to notice changes in their skin such as ne lines, wrinkles, and age spots. These signs of aging can be frustrating and lead many women to seek out treatments to help rejuvenate their skin. Intense pulsed light (IPL) treatments have become increasingly popular among women in this age group due to their ability to e ectively target a variety of skin concerns.

One of the key long-term bene ts of regular IPL treatments is the stimulation of collagen production in the skin. Collagen is a protein that helps maintain the skin's elasticity and rmness, but its production naturally decreases as we age. By undergoing regular IPL treatments, women can help to boost collagen production in their skin, leading to a more youthful and radiant complexion over time.

In addition to stimulating collagen production, IPL treatments can also help to improve the overall texture and tone of the skin. IPL targets and reduces the appearance of age spots, sun damage, and redness, resulting in a more even complexion. With continued treatments, women can expect to see a signi cant improvement in the overall quality of their skin, leading to a more youthful and rejuvenated appearance.

Another long-term bene t of regular IPL treatments is the reduction of ne lines and wrinkles. IPL works by targeting the deeper layers of the skin where collagen and elastin are produced, helping to smooth out ne lines and wrinkles over time. With consistent treatments, women can achieve a more youthful and refreshed look without the need for invasive procedures or surgeries.

Overall, regular IPL treatments can help women in the 40+ age group achieve a more youthful and radiant complexion by stimulating collagen production, improving skin texture and tone, and reducing the appearance of ne lines and wrinkles. By incorporating IPL treatments into their skincare routine, women can enjoy long-term bene ts that will leave them looking and feeling more con dent in their skin as they age gracefully.

Chapter 6: Real Women, Real Results

Testimonials from women who have tried IPL treatments

In this subchapter, we will hear from real women who have experienced the wonders of IPL treatments in their quest for age-defying beauty. These testimonials come from women in the 40+ age group who have tried IPL treatments and seen incredible results. Their stories serve as inspiration for those considering this innovative treatment to rejuvenate their skin and turn back the hands of time.

One woman, Sarah, shared her experience with IPL treatments, saying, "I was skeptical at rst, but after just a few sessions, I noticed a signi cant improvement in the texture and tone of my skin. My ne lines and wrinkles seemed to fade away, and my complexion looked brighter and more youthful. I feel more con dent and radiant than ever before."

Another woman, Emily, raved about the results she achieved with IPL treatments, stating, "I have struggled with sun damage and age spots for years, but after undergoing IPL treatments, my skin looks clearer and more even-toned. I no longer have to rely on heavy makeup to cover up my imperfections, and I feel like I can nally embrace my natural beauty."

Laura, a busy mother in her 40s, shared her experience with IPL treatments, saying, "I don't have a lot of time for complicated skincare routines, so IPL treatments have been a game-changer for me. With just a few quick sessions, my skin looks rejuvenated and more youthful. I love the convenience and e ectiveness of IPL treatments."

For many women in the 40+ age group, IPL treatments have become a staple in their skincare routine. These testimonials highlight the transformative power of IPL treatments in combating the signs of aging and achieving age-defying beauty. If you are considering IPL treatments, let these real-life stories inspire you to take the rst step towards radiant, youthful skin.

In conclusion, the testimonials from women who have tried IPL treatments speak volumes about the e ectiveness and bene ts of this innovative skincare solution. Whether you are looking to reduce ne lines and wrinkles, even out your skin tone, or combat sun damage, IPL treatments can help you achieve your goals. Take inspiration from these real-life stories and consider incorporating IPL treatments into your skincare routine to experience the age-defying beauty that so many women in the 40+ age group have already enjoyed.

Before and after photos of IPL treatments for aging skin

As women age, many may begin to notice changes in their skin, such as ne lines, wrinkles, and age spots. Fortunately, there are advanced treatments available that can help combat these signs of aging. One popular option for rejuvenating aging skin is Intense Pulsed Light (IPL) therapy. IPL treatments utilize pulses of light to target and reduce the appearance of common skin concerns, leaving skin looking more youthful and radiant.

Before undergoing IPL treatments, it can be helpful to see some before and after photos of individuals who have undergone the procedure. These photos can provide a visual representation of the potential results that can be achieved with IPL therapy. By examining these images, women in the 40+ age group can get a better idea of how IPL treatments may bene t their own skin and help them make an informed decision about pursuing this type of cosmetic procedure.

In the before photos, women may notice signs of aging such as sun damage, uneven skin tone, and ne lines. These images can serve as a reminder of the areas of concern that IPL treatments can address. After the IPL treatments, the after photos will show improvements in the skin's texture, tone, and overall appearance. Women may observe a reduction in the appearance of age spots, smoother skin, and a more youthful complexion.

It is important for women in the 40+ age group to keep in mind that individual results may vary when it comes to IPL treatments. Factors such as skin type, the severity of the skin concerns, and the number of treatment sessions can all impact the nal outcome. However, by reviewing before and after photos of IPL treatments, women can gain a better understanding of the potential bene ts and decide if this type of therapy is right for them.

Ultimately, IPL treatments can be a valuable tool in the ght against aging skin. By examining before and after photos and consulting with a quali ed skincare professional, women in the 40+ age group can take proactive steps to rejuvenate their skin and achieve a more youthful appearance. With the science behind IPL treatments on their side, women can con dently embrace the aging process and feel empowered to enhance their natural beauty.

Chapter 7: FAQs about IPL Treatments for Women 40+

Is IPL safe for aging skin?

As women age, they often become more conscious of the changes in their skin, such as ne lines, wrinkles, and age spots. Many turn to various treatments to help combat these signs of aging, with one popular option being Intense Pulsed Light (IPL) therapy. But the question remains - is IPL safe for aging skin?

IPL therapy is a non-invasive treatment that uses high-intensity pulses of light to target speci c skin concerns, such as pigmentation, redness, and ne lines. It works by heating the targeted areas of the skin, causing the body to produce new collagen and elastin, which helps to improve skin texture and tone. While IPL is generally considered safe for all skin types, including aging skin, it is essential to consult with a quali ed practitioner before undergoing treatment.

One of the key bene ts of IPL therapy for aging skin is its ability to target multiple skin concerns simultaneously. This makes it an e cient option for women looking to address a variety of issues, such as age spots, sun damage, and uneven skin tone. Additionally, IPL treatments are typically quick and require little to no downtime, making them a convenient option for busy women in their 40s and bey o n d.

However, it is crucial to note that IPL therapy may not be suitable for everyone. Women with certain skin conditions, such as rosacea or melasma, may not be good candidates for IPL treatments. Additionally, those with darker skin tones may be at a higher risk of experiencing side e ects, such as hyperpigmentation or burns. It is essential to undergo a thorough consultation with a quali ed practitioner to determine if IPL is the right treatment option for your aging skin.

In conclusion, IPL therapy can be a safe and e ective option for women in their 40s and beyond looking to rejuvenate their aging skin. With its ability to target multiple skin concerns and minimal downtime, IPL treatments o er a convenient solution for busy women seeking to improve their skin's appearance. However, it is essential to consult with a quali ed practitioner to ensure that IPL is the right treatment option for your speci c skin concerns and needs.

How many treatments are needed for optimal results?

When it comes to achieving optimal results with IPL treatments, the number of sessions required can vary depending on individual skin concerns and goals. In general, most women in the 40+ age group will see signi cant improvements in their skin after just a few treatments. However, to achieve long-lasting results and maintain a youthful appearance, it is recommended to undergo a series of treatments spaced out over several weeks or months.

For women in their 40s and beyond, a typical IPL treatment plan may consist of anywhere from 3 to 6 sessions, with each session lasting about 20-30 minutes. These sessions are usually scheduled about 4-6 weeks apart to allow the skin to heal and regenerate in between treatments. By spacing out the treatments in this way, the skin is able to gradually improve and rejuvenate over time, resulting in smoother, rmer, and more youthful-looking skin.

It is important to keep in mind that while some women may see dramatic results after just a few sessions, others may require more treatments to achieve their desired outcomes. Factors such as skin type, sun exposure, lifestyle habits, and overall skin health can all impact the number of treatments needed for optimal results. Consulting with a skincare professional who specializes in IPL treatments can help determine the best treatment plan for individual needs and goals.

In addition to the number of treatments, it is also important to follow a consistent skincare routine and adhere to any post-treatment instructions provided by the skincare professional. This may include using gentle skincare products, wearing sunscreen daily, and avoiding excessive sun exposure to maintain the results of the IPL treatments. By following these guidelines, women in the 40+ age group can achieve long-lasting results and enjoy a more youthful and radiant complexion.

Overall, while the number of treatments needed for optimal results may vary from person to person, most women in the 40+ age group can expect to see signi cant improvements in their skin after undergoing a series of IPL treatments. By working with a skincare professional to develop a personalized treatment plan and following a proper skincare routine, women can achieve a more youthful and rejuvenated appearance that lasts for years to come.

As women age, many may nd themselves seeking out various skin care procedures to help combat the signs of aging. One popular option that has gained traction in recent years is Intense Pulsed Light (IPL) treatments. These non-invasive procedures use light energy to target and improve the appearance of skin concerns such as sun damage, age spots, and ne lines. But can IPL treatments be combined with other skin care procedures for even more dramatic results?

The short answer is yes, IPL treatments can be safely combined with other skin care procedures to enhance their e ectiveness. In fact, many dermatologists and skin care experts recommend pairing IPL with treatments such as chemical peels, microdermabrasion, or laser resurfacing for a more comprehensive approach to rejuvenating the skin. By combining di erent procedures, you can target multiple skin concerns simultaneously and achieve more noticeable results in a shorter amount of time.

When considering combining IPL treatments with other skin care procedures, it is important to consult with a quali ed dermatologist or skin care professional. They can assess your skin type and speci c concerns to develop a customized treatment plan that is safe and e ective for you. Additionally, they can provide guidance on the timing and spacing of treatments to ensure optimal results and minimize the risk of any adverse e ects.

One popular combination is the pairing of IPL treatments with microneedling, a procedure that uses tiny needles to create micro-injuries in the skin, stimulating collagen production and improving skin texture. When used in conjunction with IPL, microneedling can enhance the penetration of light energy and promote even better results in terms of skin tightening and rejuvenation.

In conclusion, combining IPL treatments with other skin care procedures can be a powerful way to address multiple skin concerns and achieve more dramatic results. By working with a quali ed professional to develop a personalized treatment plan, women in the 40+ age group can take advantage of the synergistic e ects of di erent procedures to rejuvenate their skin and achieve a more youthful appearance. Remember to always prioritize safety and consult with a professional before embarking on any skin care regimen.

Chapter 8: Finding the Right IPL Provider

Questions to ask when choosing an IPL provider

When it comes to choosing an IPL provider for your skin treatments, there are several important questions you should ask to ensure you are making the best decision for your skin and overall well-being. First and foremost, inquire about the quali cations and experience of the IPL provider. It is crucial to choose a provider who is trained and certi ed in performing IPL treatments, as this will ensure that you receive safe and e ective care.

Another important question to ask is what type of IPL device the provider uses. Di erent IPL devices have varying levels of e ectiveness and safety, so it is essential to choose a provider who uses a high-quality and reputable device. Additionally, ask about the provider's experience in using the speci c IPL device they use, as this can impact the results you achieve from your treatments.

It is also important to inquire about the provider's approach to treatment planning and customization. Every individual's skin is unique, and a one-size- ts-all approach to IPL treatments may not be e ective or safe. Ask the provider how they assess your skin and develop a customized treatment plan that addresses your speci c concerns and goals.

Furthermore, ask about the potential risks and side e ects of IPL treatments, as well as how the provider mitigates these risks. A reputable provider will be transparent about the potential risks associated with IPL treatments and will have protocols in place to minimize these risks and ensure your safety.

Lastly, inquire about the provider's follow-up care and support. IPL treatments often require multiple sessions for optimal results, so it is important to choose a provider who o ers comprehensive follow-up care to monitor your progress and address any concerns that may arise. By asking these important questions when choosing an IPL provider, you can make an informed decision that will help you achieve beautiful, age-defying skin.

Researching the credentials and experience of IPL practitioners

When considering undergoing Intense Pulsed Light (IPL) treatments, it is crucial to thoroughly research the credentials and experience of the practitioners who will be administering the procedures. As women in the 40+ age group, it is important to prioritize the safety and e ectiveness of any beauty treatments we undergo. By taking the time to ensure that the IPL practitioner is well-trained and experienced in performing these treatments, we can feel more con dent in the results we will achieve. One of the rst steps in researching the credentials of an IPL practitioner is to inquire about their training and certi cation in performing IPL treatments. Look for practitioners who have received formal training in the use of IPL devices and have obtained certi cations from reputable organizations. Additionally, ask about their experience level in performing IPL treatments speci cally for women in the 40+ age group. Experience plays a signi cant role in the success of IPL treatments, as practitioners who have treated a variety of skin types and conditions are more likely to achieve optimal results.

Another important aspect to consider when researching IPL practitioners is to inquire about their track record of successful treatments. Ask for before-and-after photos of previous clients who are in a similar age group and have similar skin concerns. This will give you a better idea of the practitioner's skill level and the potential outcomes you can expect from the IPL treatments. Additionally, consider reading reviews and testimonials from past clients to gauge their satisfaction with the results and overall experience with the practitioner.

In addition to researching the credentials and experience of IPL practitioners, it is also important to ensure that the facility where the treatments will be performed adheres to strict safety and hygiene standards. Look for a clean and well-maintained facility that uses state-of-the-art IPL devices and follows proper sterilization protocols. By choosing a reputable facility with high standards of care, you can minimize the risk of complications and achieve the best possible results from your IPL treatments.

Overall, researching the credentials and experience of IPL practitioners is essential for women in the 40+ age group who are considering undergoing these treatments. By taking the time to vet potential practitioners, we can ensure that we are in capable hands and increase the likelihood of achieving our desired results. Remember to prioritize safety, experience, and client satisfaction when choosing an IPL practitioner, and don't hesitate to ask questions and seek out additional information before committing to any treatments.

When considering undergoing IPL treatments, it is important for women in the 40+ age group to take cost into consideration. IPL treatments can vary in price depending on the area being treated, the number of sessions required, and the expertise of the provider. It is essential to research di erent providers and compare prices to ensure you are getting the best value for your money.

One cost consideration for IPL treatments is the location of the provider. Providers in urban areas tend to charge higher prices compared to those in rural areas. However, it is important to weigh the cost savings against the convenience and quality of care provided by the provider. Additionally, some providers o er package deals or discounts for multiple sessions, which can help lower the overall cost of t reat men t .

Another factor to consider when determining the cost of IPL treatments is the size of the treatment area. Larger areas, such as the legs or back, will typically cost more than smaller areas like the face or underarms. Be sure to discuss the speci c areas you would like to have treated with your provider to get an accurate estimate of the cost.

It is also important to factor in the number of sessions required for optimal results when considering the cost of IPL treatments. Some women may see results after just one session, while others may require multiple sessions to achieve their desired outcome. Discussing your goals with your provider will help determine the number of sessions needed and the associated cost.

Overall, while cost is an important consideration when undergoing IPL treatments, it is essential to prioritize the quality of care and expertise of the provider. Investing in a reputable provider may cost more upfront but can lead to better results and a more satisfying experience in the long run. Be sure to research di erent providers, compare prices, and discuss your goals with your provider to ensure you are making an informed decision about your IPL treatments.

Chapter 9: Embracing Age-Defying Beauty with IPL

The psychological bene ts of looking and feeling younger

As women age, it is natural to want to maintain a youthful appearance both physically and mentally. One way to achieve this is through IPL treatments, which can help improve the overall look and feel of your skin. But beyond the physical bene ts, there are also psychological advantages to looking and feeling younger that should not be overlooked.

One of the key psychological bene ts of looking and feeling younger is increased self-con dence. When you are happy with your appearance, you are more likely to feel good about yourself and exude con dence in all areas of your life. This can lead to improved relationships, career success, and overall well-being. IPL treatments can help you achieve a more youthful appearance, which in turn can boost your self-esteem and con dence.

Another psychological bene t of looking and feeling younger is a positive outlook on life. When you are happy with how you look, you are more likely to have a positive attitude and outlook on life. This can lead to increased happiness, improved mental health, and a greater sense of overall well-being. IPL treatments can help you achieve a more youthful appearance, which can help improve your mood and outlook on life.

Furthermore, looking and feeling younger can also lead to increased motivation and energy levels. When you feel good about yourself, you are more likely to take care of yourself and stay active. This can lead to increased energy levels, improved physical health, and a greater sense of motivation to achieve your goals. IPL treatments can help you look and feel younger, which can in turn lead to increased motivation and energy levels to tackle whatever challenges come your way.

In addition, looking and feeling younger can also help you feel more connected to your inner self. When you are happy with your appearance, you are more likely to feel comfortable in your own skin and at peace with yourself. This can lead to a greater sense of self-acceptance, self-love, and self-con dence. IPL treatments can help you achieve a more youthful appearance, which can help you feel more connected to your inner self and at peace with who you are.

Overall, the psychological bene ts of looking and feeling younger are numerous and should not be underestimated. By investing in IPL treatments to achieve a more youthful appearance, women in the 40+ age group can experience increased self-con dence, a positive outlook on life, improved motivation and energy levels, and a greater sense of connection to their inner selves. Embracing age-defying beauty through IPL treatments can have a profound impact on both your physical and psychological well-being, leading to a happier, more ful lling life.

Maintaining confidence and self-esteem as you age

As women age, it's common to experience uctuations in con dence and self-esteem. This can be due to a variety of factors, including changes in physical appearance, health concerns, or societal pressures. However, it's important to remember that con dence and self-esteem are not solely based on external factors, but also on how we perceive ourselves and our abilities.

One way to maintain con dence and self-esteem as you age is by taking care of your skin. Intense pulsed light (IPL) treatments are a popular option for women in their 40s and beyond, as they can help reduce the appearance of age spots, sun damage, and ne lines. By investing in your skin's health, you can boost your con dence and feel more comfortable in your own skin.

In addition to skincare treatments like IPL, it's important to practice self-care and prioritize your mental and emotional well-being. This can include engaging in activities that bring you joy, surrounding yourself with positive in uences, and seeking support from friends and loved ones. By taking care of yourself holistically, you can build a strong foundation for con dence and self-esteem.

Another key aspect of maintaining con dence and self-esteem as you age is embracing your uniqueness and celebrating your achievements. Remember that beauty comes in all shapes, sizes, and ages, and that there is no one-size- ts-all de nition of beauty. By focusing on your strengths and accomplishments, you can boost your self-esteem and feel empowered to take on new challenges.

Ultimately, con dence and self-esteem are a journey, not a destination. By incorporating skincare treatments like IPL, practicing self-care, and embracing your individuality, you can feel more con dent and self-assured as you age. Remember that you are worthy of love and respect, no matter your age, and that your beauty shines from within.

Embracing the aging process with grace and positivity

As women age, it is natural for our bodies to go through changes, including the appearance of wrinkles, age spots, and other signs of aging. However, embracing the aging process with grace and positivity can help us navigate these changes with con dence and self-assurance. Intense pulsed light (IPL) treatments o er a non-invasive and e ective way to address these common signs of aging, helping women in the 40+ age group maintain their youthful appearance.

One key aspect of embracing the aging process with grace and positivity is accepting and celebrating the wisdom and experience that come with age. Instead of viewing wrinkles and age spots as aws to be hidden or corrected, women in the 40+ age group can choose to see them as symbols of a life well-lived. By embracing these signs of aging, women can cultivate a sense of inner beauty and con dence that radiates from within.

IPL treatments can play a signi cant role in helping women in the 40+ age group maintain their youthful appearance and boost their self-con dence. By targeting areas of concern such as sun damage, age spots, and ne lines, IPL treatments can improve skin tone and texture, resulting in a more youthful and radiant complexion. Embracing these treatments as part of a comprehensive skincare routine can empower women to take control of their aging process and feel con dent in their skin.

In addition to the physical bene ts of IPL treatments, embracing the aging process with grace and positivity can also have a positive impact on mental and emotional well-being. By choosing to focus on self-acceptance and self-love, women in the 40+ age group can cultivate a sense of inner peace and contentment that transcends the super cial aspects of aging. This holistic approach to aging can lead to a greater sense of overall well-being and ful llment.

In conclusion, embracing the aging process with grace and positivity is a powerful way for women in the 40+ age group to navigate the inevitable changes that come with getting older. By incorporating IPL treatments into their skincare routine and adopting a mindset of self-acceptance and self-love, women can enhance their natural beauty and embrace their age with con dence and grace. Age-defying beauty is not about defying the passage of time, but rather about embracing it with grace and positivity.

www.ingramcontent.com/pod-product-compliance
Lightning Source LLC
Chambersburg PA
CBHW080052270726
48653CB00045B/3910